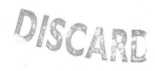

The First Woman Doctor

By
**Antonia
Goodspeed**

A CPI GROUP Book
from
SRA

Art and Photo Credits

Art: Cindy Spencer
Photo: page 46, Courtesy of New York Downtown Hospital

Library of Congress Catalog Card Number: 92-45996

Library of Congress Cataloging in Publication Data

Goodspeed, Antonia.
  The first woman doctor / by Antonia Goodspeed.

  p. cm. — (Famous Firsts)
  SUMMARY: Presents the life story of Elizabeth Blackwell, who, during the mid-1800s, became the first woman doctor in the United States, despite problems and opposition.

  ISBN 0-383-03820-0

  1. Blackwell, Elizabeth, 1821–1910 — Juvenile literature.
  2. Women physicians — United States — Biography — Juvenile literature. [1. Blackwell, Elizabeth, 1821–1910. 2. Women physicians. 3. Physicians] I. Title. II. Series

R154.B623G66   1994
610'.92 — dc20   92-45996
[B]   CIP
                                                            AC

Manufactured in the United States of America

Product Code 87-003820

ISBN 0-383-03820-0

CONTENTS

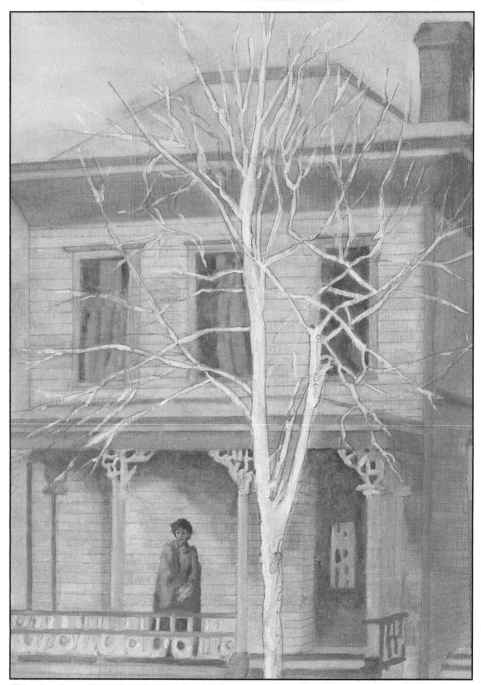

Elizabeth walked back and forth along the porch that evening. What was to become of her? What should she do with her life?

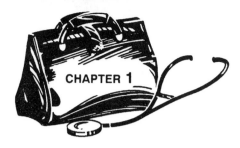

A Promise to a Friend

It should have been a pleasant evening at home with her family. But Elizabeth did not join in the conversation. Nor could she concentrate on reading. So many thoughts crowded into her mind. Too restless to sit near the warm fire, she grabbed a cape and rushed out into the cold winter night.

As she paced along the porch, Elizabeth Blackwell reviewed her life. She was 24 years old and well educated for a young woman of the mid-1800s. She read German and books on philosophy. Through her writer friend, Harriet Beecher Stowe, she knew many interesting people in Cincinnati society. She was interested in the great issues of her time. By working with the Anti-Slavery Society, she was helping people who had escaped from slavery.

But what was to become of her? What should she do with her life? Elizabeth thought about marriage. In those days, however, married women were considered less important than their husbands. Elizabeth would never marry a man who did not treat her as an equal. She had been teaching for a few years. Yet she did not want to be a teacher for the rest of her life. She wanted to give all her energy to an important cause. But what kind of work would it be? The answer would come in a surprising way.

At this time, a friend of the Blackwells', Mary Donaldson, was dying of cancer. When Elizabeth visited her, Mary spoke about her illness. She had a type of cancer that affected only women. The suffering was terrible. Mary knew that other women suffered in the same way.

She told Elizabeth who her doctor was. She shook her head slowly and moaned. "Oh, Elizabeth. Men just cannot understand women's sicknesses. If only I could find a woman doctor." But, there were no woman doctors in the United States in the middle of the nineteenth century. All doctors were men.

"You are young and strong, my dear," Mary went on. "You have a keen mind and like to study. Why don't you try to become a doctor?"

Elizabeth was stunned. Become a doctor? What a foolish idea! She was amazed by the very thought. Besides, the sight of blood and sores made Elizabeth squirm.

"Please, my dear," Mary pleaded in a faint voice. "Promise me you will at least think about it." Weak as she was, Mary held Elizabeth's hands tightly. After a long time, Elizabeth whispered, "I promise."

Mary Donaldson died not long after their talk. But Elizabeth did not forget her promise. She thought about what it would mean to become a

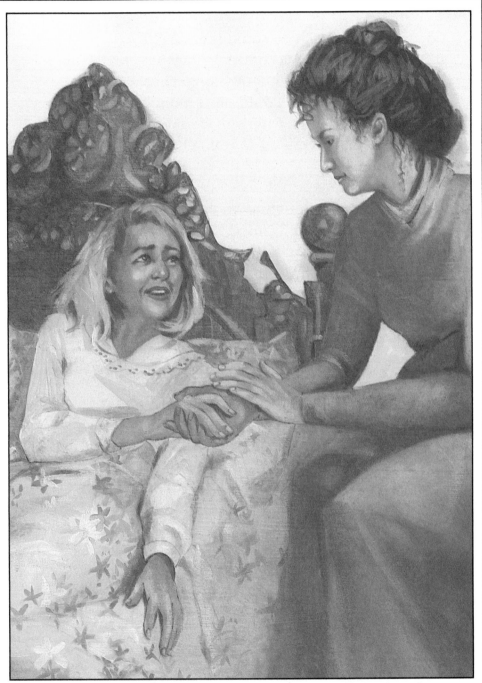

Her dying friend, Mary, urged Elizabeth to become a doctor in order to help other women who suffered this way.

doctor. At first, all she could see were the difficulties. She would have to leave her comfortable life. She would have to study subjects she had always avoided. She would need money to pay for that education. Above all, she would need the courage to do something that no other woman had done before.

Certainly, she could not doubt that Mary's view of men doctors was right. Women doctors could be of great help to other women. They could bring sympathy and understanding to women patients in ways that men never could.

Elizabeth did not make her decision quickly. And before she did, she talked with her family. Her brother Henry was delighted. "If anyone can do it, our Elizabeth can!" he encouraged.

Could Elizabeth Blackwell become the first woman doctor? She wasn't certain, but she was resolved to try.

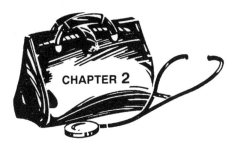

CHAPTER 2

Samuel Blackwell Speaks Out

Elizabeth Blackwell was born in Bristol, England, on February 3, 1821. She was the third child of Hannah and Samuel Blackwell. There would be six other children after her. The Blackwell home also had room for Samuel's four sisters.

Religion was a big part of their family life. So were picnics, long walks in the country, and reading books and poetry. Samuel Blackwell's business was growing sugar cane and selling the processed sugar. He was so prosperous that he could afford to have all his children educated at home by private tutors. Samuel had strong ideas about education. His ideas were not always shared by other family members. The children were used to hearing their father discuss his opinions with Aunt Bar, the sternest of his sisters.

"Sheer nonsense, brother Samuel!" she would say. "What possible use can your daughters make of all this education?"

"My daughters have as good minds as my sons, and I see no reason why they should not be taught to use them in the same way. As to what use they will put them in later life, that will be for them to decide."

Most English children were sent to their rooms when visitors came. But the Blackwells allowed their children to listen to the writers, missionaries, and people in government who visited them.

Samuel disagreed with some ideas of the time. His sugar business depended on the slaves who worked on the sugar-cane plantations of Caribbean islands. But Samuel believed that slavery was wrong. He wanted to find a way to keep his business while ending the injustice of slavery.

First, Samuel Blackwell had to face another problem. In 1831, England was going through very hard times. There had been years of poor harvests. Many people were out of work. There were unjust laws and taxes, and many people were dissatisfied with their lives. Finally, riots broke out. In Bristol, public buildings were burned. The townspeople fought with police in the streets.

When the riots were over, Elizabeth knew her happy childhood had ended, too. Sugar prices fell and the Blackwells were in danger of losing their business. Samuel was too proud to borrow money. Instead, he sold his house and his company. In August of 1832, when Elizabeth was 11, the Blackwell family set sail for America. They would make new lives for themselves in the New World.

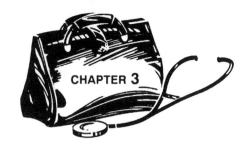

CHAPTER 3

Starting Over

When the Blackwells arrived in New York City they found it almost deserted. An outbreak of a terrible disease called cholera had caused many people to flee to the countryside.

The New York City the Blackwells found in the 1830s was dirty and badly lighted. The roads were wide but poorly paved. The hotels were shabby compared with those in England. There were no grand buildings like those of English cities. There were no quaint villages in the countryside.

Yet, New York was an exciting place. People from all parts of the world had settled there. They had fascinating stories to tell about their homelands. They worked hard to make new lives in a new land. There was talk of getting voting reforms, better wages, and improved working conditions.

Again, Samuel Blackwell became involved with the issue of slavery. With so much land in America, he reasoned, why not encourage freed slaves to grow sugar crops? Then, slave labor could be stopped. Other businessmen resisted his ideas. After all, why should they change things when business was going so well?

Hannah Blackwell and the children also worked for the antislavery cause, selling food and crafts to support the movement. Two of Elizabeth's older sisters opened a school for black children. After a while, the large, active family moved to a bigger house in Jersey City, New Jersey. Elizabeth, now 14, traveled by ferry across the Hudson River to school in New York. She and her sisters went to lectures and antislavery meetings. She enjoyed her teenage years, but growing up was not always easy. She sometimes felt out of place in her own family. Her sister Marianne was very popular and more at ease with people than Elizabeth was. All her brothers were popular, as well. She felt left out when visits to friends and relatives were planned. Elizabeth felt closest to her father. She wished she could be more like him. He was so warm and friendly, yet strong and secure.

There was always much going on at home. Elizabeth was studying music, and she practiced piano for several hours every day. She also enjoyed long walks with her brother, Sam, in good weather or bad. But soon all the members of the Blackwell family would be touched by very serious problems.

One night in December 1835, fire swept through lower Manhattan. Building after building went up in flames. While the family watched the flames helplessly from across the river in Jersey City, Samuel rushed to New York to try to protect his

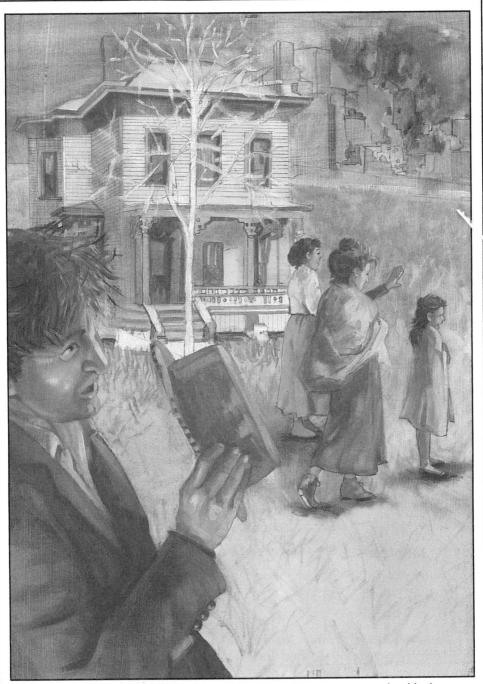

The Blackwell family helplessly watched the flames across the Hudson river, hoping their father's sugar warehouses would be spared.

sugar warehouses. Three days later he came home. Forty blocks of the city were gone, but his sugar warehouses were safe!

The family's relief, however, did not last long. Within a year, another fire did destroy one of the warehouses. With the loss of much of their income, the Blackwells had to change their lives. Hannah let the servants go. The older girls took turns doing the housework. Elizabeth gave up her music lessons. Anna took a job as a music teacher in Vermont. There were no new clothes or birthday presents. For Elizabeth, the worst change was the one she saw in her father. His fun-loving spirit was lost.

He spoke to no one about his plans for the future. Would they return to England? Would they stay near New York? Could the sugar business be saved? If Samuel knew the answer to those questions, he was not telling the rest of the family.

But Samuel Blackwell was not beaten by his loss. He began to study the progress being made in Europe in getting sugar from sugar beets. And when a cousin returned from the West, Samuel listened to his stories. The American West was a land of opportunity. Samuel could be the first to open a sugar company in the West.

Suddenly, Samuel's spirit returned. With new enthusiasm, he traveled West to see for himself. When he returned, he was eager to move. So in May of 1838, the family began another journey. This time they were headed for the frontier.

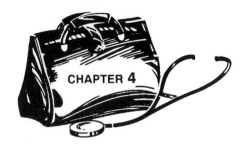

CHAPTER 4

A Tragedy and a Decision

As the side-wheeler steamed along the Ohio River, the Blackwells got their first look at Cincinnati. The streets and waterfront were bustling. Neat brick houses dotted the hills. What a wonderful surprise this frontier city was!

Samuel soon found a large house for his family, and a building for his business. For a few months, things looked hopeful. Then, suddenly, Samuel became sick and died. The family — especially Elizabeth — missed him deeply. But there was little time for sadness. The family found there was only $20 in the bank, and many bills to pay.

In great need of money, the women turned to what they knew best — teaching. Aunt Mary, Anna, Marianne, and Elizabeth opened a school for neighborhood children. Elizabeth, at 17, was not happy as a teacher.

"I was afraid of my pupils," she later confessed. "I controlled them only by steady quietness, which they took for sternness, but which was really fear."

In the years that followed, the sisters would talk

about what they would really like to do. They also talked about the jobs that were open to women. Jobs in factories, as servants, seamstresses, teachers — the opportunities were few. Still, there were some small signs of change. In 1833, Oberlin College had opened in Ohio. It was the first college to admit men and women of all races. In 1837, Mount Holyoke opened to educate women in many professions.

By 1844, brothers Henry and Sam had well-paying jobs. The Blackwell women were able to close their school. Anna left to teach in a school in New York. But what was there for Elizabeth to do? She did not want to depend on her family. She had to find a way to do something for society. So when the offer of a teaching job came along, Elizabeth took it.

The people of Henderson, Kentucky, were friendly to the new teacher. The students were pleasant, too, and Elizabeth was happy for a while. But Kentucky was a slave state. For the first time, Elizabeth could see for herself the cruelty of slavery. It was no longer just a topic at an antislavery meeting. Here were real people being treated savagely. At the end of the term, Elizabeth left Kentucky and returned home.

Back in Cincinnati, Elizabeth joined her family's new group of friends. She especially admired Harriet Beecher Stowe. Here was a woman who combined her career as a writer with the responsibilities of a large family.

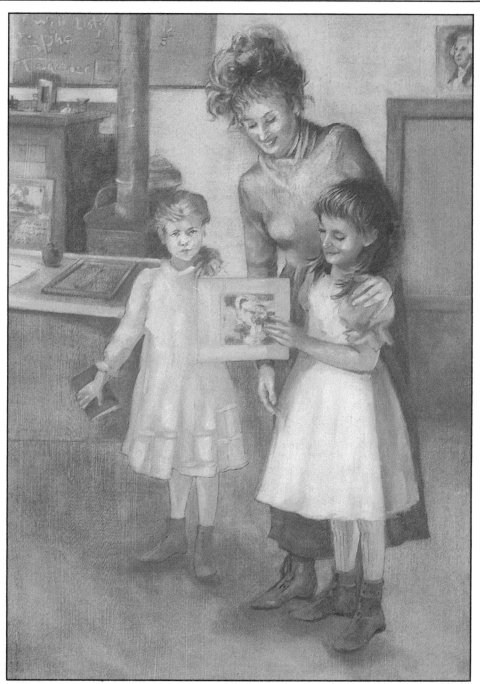

Elizabeth enjoyed teaching her students in Kentucky, but she was dismayed by the cruelty of slavery in the state.

At Harriet's literary club, Elizabeth met a man she became very fond of. He was educated and interesting. He began walking her home from meetings and sending her flowers. When Elizabeth showed him her latest book on philosophy, he suggested she read poetry instead.

He once said to her, "You shouldn't be bothering that pretty little head about social theories that no woman could possibly understand. Better to leave the reforming of society to us men, who have the responsibility of running the world."

It was no surprise to hear a man talk that way. Elizabeth knew that many men felt that women's duty was to make life easier for men. Then men could carry out the important work in life. But she was disappointed to learn that *this* man thought that way, too.

It was after this that Elizabeth found herself pacing the porch on a cold winter's night. By the coming spring, Mary Donaldson's idea would rarely be out of Elizabeth's mind. The decision took a long time. Yes! She would try to become a doctor!

But if making the decision was difficult, reaching her goal would take all the courage Elizabeth Blackwell had.

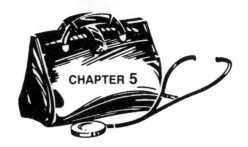

The First Difficult Steps

Once the decision had been made, Elizabeth acted quickly. She knew what had to be done. She must go to medical school. And she had to find a way to pay for her studies.

Elizabeth spoke to her friend, Harriet Beecher Stowe. A worthy idea, Harriet agreed, but not practical. But she promised to speak to a famous Cincinnati doctor about Elizabeth's plan. His reaction was harsh. No medical school would accept a woman. Elizabeth would hear that same reaction, again and again, from every doctor she spoke to.

But she was not defeated. When her sister, Anna, told her about a teaching job in North Carolina, Elizabeth accepted. This job could be a way around her problem. The principal of the school, John Dickson, was a doctor. While she worked at his school, Elizabeth could study his medical books. She could begin her education on her own!

As she had planned, Elizabeth taught during the day and read medical books at night. She even took time to open a school for the children of slaves. Since it was against the law in North Carolina to teach slaves how to read and write, Elizabeth taught the children stories from the Bible.

Elizabeth was earning money and learning at the same time. But progress was slow. When would her dream of becoming a doctor come true? Then, John Dickson decided to close his school. For a while, Elizabeth's hopes seemed to vanish. If she couldn't find another job, she would have to leave North Carolina and postpone her education.

It was Mrs. Dickson who found a solution. Elizabeth could travel with her to Charleston, South Carolina. There, she could live in the home of Samuel Dickson, John's brother. Samuel, also a doctor, could help her with her education.

Elizabeth impressed Dr. Dickson with her determination. He taught her Greek and outlined a course of study for her. He also helped her find a job teaching music. In the meantime, Elizabeth continued writing to doctors, telling them of her plan. One of the few who answered was a Dr. Warrington of Philadelphia. He reminded her of the difficulties that lay ahead. If she wanted to help the sick, surely being a nurse would be easier. But, if she came to Philadelphia, he would see her.

Thinking only of that one hopeful note in his letter, Elizabeth went to Philadelphia. The city had several medical schools. But even letters from Dr. Warrington could not open the doors to a woman. The only college that would allow Elizabeth to attend

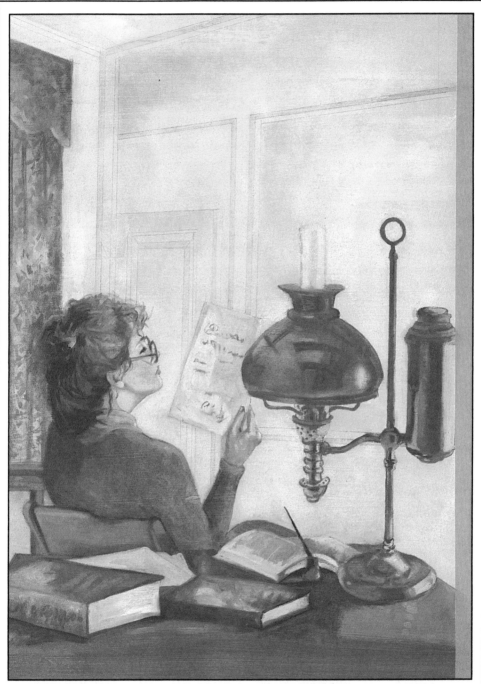

Elizabeth had written to many doctors. Dr. Warrington, one of the few who responded, agreed to see her if she would come to Philadelphia.

required that she cut her hair and dress like a man!

Dr. Warrington did help Elizabeth in an important way. He introduced her to a Dr. Allen, who accepted her into his private school of anatomy. Until now, the only anatomy Elizabeth had learned was the anatomy of a beetle that she had once dissected. Just looking at anatomical diagrams of human beings in medical books made her sick. But now, with Dr. Allen's sensitive and patient teaching, Elizabeth became fascinated by the study of the human body. In fact, she made up her mind to become a surgeon.

Elizabeth still had to graduate from a medical school for her plan to succeed. She wrote to medical schools throughout the East, waiting impatiently for each answer. Twenty-eight replies. Each the same. No. No. No.

Then, in October of 1847, came a different answer. It was from Geneva Medical College in upper New York State. The students of the school had voted. All were in favor of admitting her! At last, a tremendous weight dropped from her shoulders. All her efforts and those of her friends had paid off. She immediately accepted the offer.

When Elizabeth arrived in Geneva, she was proud and happy. She would work hard to be the first woman to be graduated from Geneva Medical College. But she would have been shocked to learn how she came to be accepted.

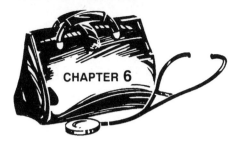

CHAPTER 6

The Joke
That Failed

The head of Geneva Medical College had not known what to do. Here was a letter from Dr. Warrington, recommending a student to his school. Ordinarily, he would have agreed right away. But this student was a woman. He didn't want to offend the important doctor. But he certainly was not ready to accept a woman. What would people think? How would the students react? It took weeks before he came up with a way out. He decided to have the students vote on admitting Elizabeth.

The voting was treated as a joke. Although the students voted for Elizabeth, they really didn't believe a woman would show up for medical school. If she did, they would enjoy teasing her and watching her reaction.

But Elizabeth did show up. When she arrived, the people in town stared and whispered behind her back. *What respectable woman would want to study medicine? Perhaps she is crazy. Watch her for signs of violence.*

The students at the college had a different

impression. Elizabeth was small, quiet, and calm.
The men did not carry on in their usual, noisy way
when she attended class. They seemed to be more
serious about their studies when she was around.

Elizabeth was usually too busy to notice how the
men reacted to her. She studied hard — often
working until midnight — in order to catch up on
the lectures she had missed at the beginning of
the term.

Dr. Webster, the anatomy professor, became
Elizabeth's strongest supporter. He encouraged her
to become a surgeon. Elizabeth learned so much
from his dissection classes that she wrote in her
diary, "Oh, this is the way to learn!"

But when the class was to study the organs of
reproduction, even Dr. Webster's support seemed to
fail. He was afraid of how the other students would
react. Every time this topic was covered, the men
disturbed the lecture with jokes and laughter. He
asked Elizabeth not to attend the class.

Elizabeth was hurt, but she was angry as well.
She wrote Dr. Webster a letter. "I am a serious
student," she wrote. "I have a right to the same
information and experience as all the other
students. But, if everyone agrees that my presence
would be embarrassing, I will not attend."

Dr. Webster read the letter to the class. Once
again, the men voted in her favor. As Elizabeth
walked to her seat, the men were silent. During the
class session, she had to keep from smiling. The
men were trying so hard to behave. Years later,

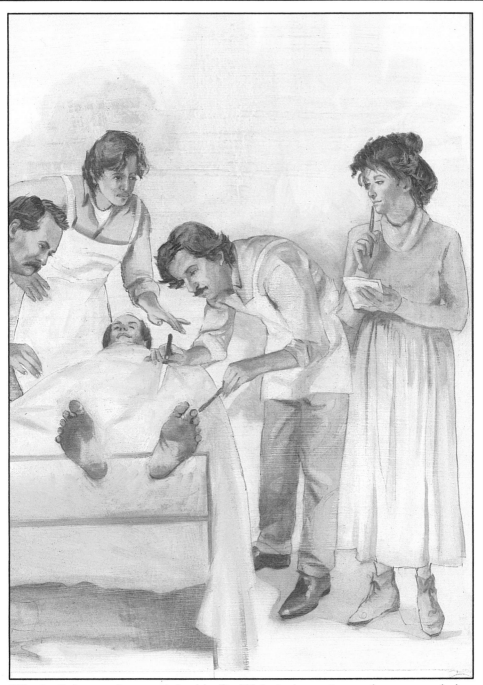

Elizabeth learned a great deal in Dr. Webster's anatomy classes, and she was encouraged when he suggested that she become a surgeon.

Stephen Smith, a friend and fellow student, would remember that day. No one was telling the usual jokes. For the first time, the students actually listened to the lecture and learned something.

That day was an important one for Elizabeth. She was no longer the "lady medical student." Now she was simply another student — and a good one at that.

But being accepted at Geneva was only a beginning. At the end of her first term, Elizabeth looked for work that would give her some practical experience. She was able to find a job at Blockley, a hospital for the poor in Philadelphia. None of the doctors wanted her there. And not all the female patients were happy about Elizabeth either. The idea of a woman caring for them in the hospital was new and strange.

Blockley was a grim place. Many poor, sick, and dying people were crowded into its huge wards. But, for the first time, Elizabeth was helping sick people. She was doing things she had only read about at Geneva.

The work became more pressing when typhus broke out in the area. Many people with this deadly, contagious disease were sent to Blockley to be treated. Later, Elizabeth would write about what she had learned. Her experience also helped her form ideas that would be important to her for the rest of her life. Fresh air, sunshine, cleanliness, and exercise, she felt, could help prevent sickness. She did not realize that by expressing these simple

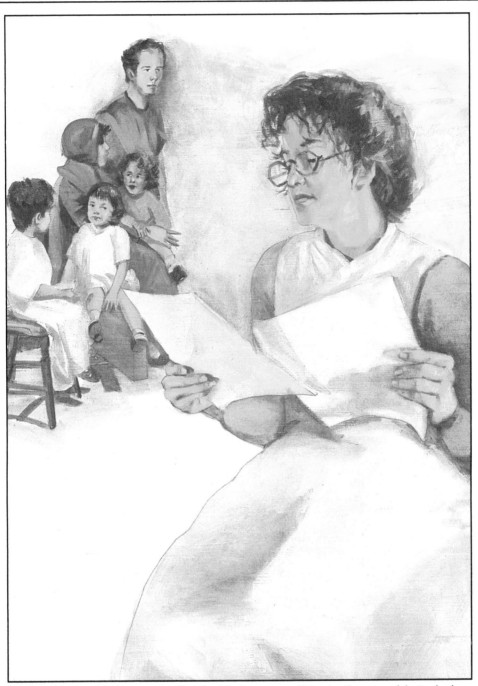

At Blockley, with its wards filled with the poor, Elizabeth was able to help sick people for the first time, doing things she had only read about before.

ideas, she was far ahead of her time.

In the fall, Elizabeth returned to Geneva. She had to complete another term of study before she could work as a doctor. Then, she would have to pass her examinations. As usual, Elizabeth put all her energies to the task. She had come so far. She would not fail now.

On January 23, 1849, Elizabeth Blackwell graduated from Geneva Medical College. Her brother, Harry, was there to see her accept her diploma. Her fellow students applauded her. Doctors made speeches. People lined up in the street to see her. But Elizabeth was so proud she hardly noticed. She had kept her promise to Mary Donaldson. Elizabeth Blackwell had become a doctor.

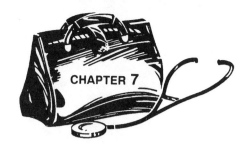

CHAPTER 7

Is Everything Lost?

The joy that Elizabeth felt at graduation did not last long. She was a doctor in name only as long as she couldn't work as one. No hospital would offer her a job. If she could not work in America, she decided, she would go to France. Great advances were being made in the hospitals of Paris.

But the only place in Paris that would accept her was La Maternité. It was a hospital where women went to have their babies. For three months, Elizabeth lived and worked alongside the French women who wanted to become midwives. She was allowed only to watch the deliveries and the operations. Even though she was a doctor, she was treated like a student.

Nevertheless, Elizabeth decided to stay for another three months. It was a decision that would change her life.

Early one November morning, Elizabeth was treating a baby with a serious eye infection. While she rinsed the baby's eyes, some of the liquid splashed into her own left eye. She washed her eye

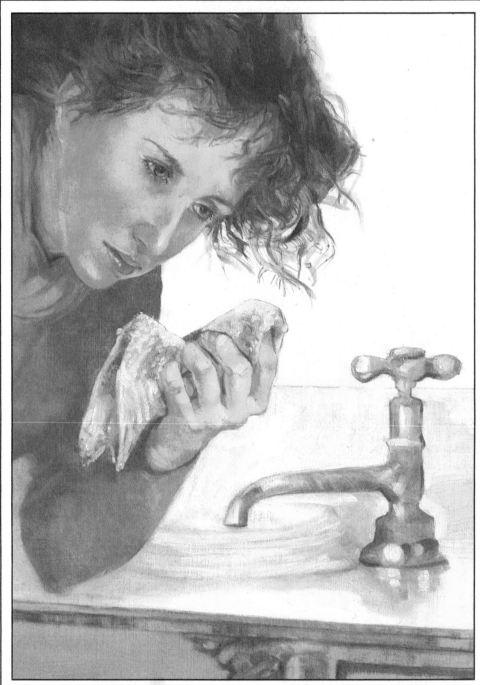

Elizabeth washed her eye in order to prevent an infection, but she contracted a disease that would leave her blind in one eye.

and worked for the rest of the day. By the evening, her eye was swollen and painful. She couldn't ignore it any longer. She had contracted the eye disease — a disease that could lead to blindness.

For days, she was treated every two hours. The treatments were painful and left her weak and shaken. Could doctors save the sight in her left eye? Would the infection spread to the other eye?

After three weeks, Elizabeth was able to open her right eye. The infection had not spread. But she was nearly blind in her left eye. For months, she went from hope to sorrow. Her right eye grew stronger. But when she tried to read, the pain in her left eye returned. She wanted to believe that she could overcome this setback as she had earlier setbacks.

While she grew stronger, she received a letter that lifted her spirits. St. Bartholomew's Hospital in London agreed to admit her as a student. Now, Elizabeth had to face the hardest choice of her life. Blind in one eye, she could never be a surgeon. Should she give up her dream of working as a doctor? Then, she remembered the filthy wards of Blockley. She could see again the suffering in the operating rooms of La Maternité. There was still a great deal of work Elizabeth Blackwell could do.

In November of 1850, fitted with a glass eye, Elizabeth arrived in London. But one area of medicine was not open to her at St. Bartholomew's. The professor of women's diseases did not approve of women becoming doctors. So, Elizabeth

Blackwell — a doctor — could not hear lectures on women's diseases.

Still, Elizabeth added to her practical knowledge of medicine. She also began to question some of the treatments and practices that were common at the time. She felt simple cleanliness could prevent some kinds of diseases. Perhaps some of the fevers and deaths that followed operations were caused by the filthy conditions in the operating rooms.

In England, Elizabeth met many young women who admired her. She was working in a profession that had been reserved for men. She had gone beyond the limits that held back most English women of the time. One such woman was Florence Nightingale. Florence longed to leave the comfort of her wealthy home and become a nurse. Her family was shocked at the idea. They did not even approve of Florence's friendship with Elizabeth.

Florence tried to persuade Elizabeth to stay in England. The two women could open their own hospital. Unlike all the others, it would be roomy, full of fresh air and sunlight. And it would be clean. But Elizabeth knew that England was still not ready to accept a woman doctor. Perhaps now America would be.

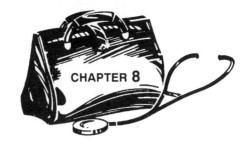

CHAPTER 8

Dr. Blackwell Moves In

Miss Elizabeth Blackwell, M.D., has just
opened an office at Number 44, University
Place, and is prepared to practice in every
department of her profession.

After this advertisement appeared in the New
York Tribune, Elizabeth waited for patients. No one
came. Her landlady was suspicious of her. People
in the street avoided her or shouted at her. She got
threatening letters in the mail. Were the people of
New York going to reject her?

Alone in her office, with little to do, Elizabeth
began to write down her ideas about health and
about how to prevent disease. Then, she hit upon a
plan. In order to get these ideas to the public, she
would deliver them herself.

She sold tickets to lectures she called "The Laws
of Life, with Special Reference to the Physical
Education of Girls." She spoke in the basement of a
church. Much of what she said then is common
sense today. But in 1852, these talks about the
human body were shocking to most women. Those
who stayed to listen became Elizabeth's first patients.

Elizabeth's younger sister, Emily, joined her in New York. Emily, too, wanted to study medicine. Now, she was trying to get into a medical school. Many schools turned her down — even Geneva, where Elizabeth had gotten her degree.

Both sisters eagerly read a new book about slavery. *Uncle Tom's Cabin* was written by their friend, Harriet Beecher Stowe, who was now a famous writer. There was other good news as well. Emily was accepted into Rush Medical College in Chicago.

With Emily away at school, Elizabeth was alone. She did not have enough patients to keep her busy. She looked for a job at a clinic. Once again, the responses were the same. There were no jobs for women. Elizabeth, angry at being turned down, decided to open her own clinic. It would be a place where poor people would be treated without charge.

At first the patients didn't trust a woman doctor. But the clinic was filled after word of Elizabeth's skill and kindness got around. Elizabeth also visited patients in their homes. She felt the terrible conditions in the tenements must be helping to spread disease.

Elizabeth's life never seemed to be free of troubles. Emily, she learned, had to find a new school. Rush Medical College no longer wanted a female medical student. Meanwhile, Elizabeth's landlady was still hostile toward her. Using money borrowed from friends, Elizabeth bought her own house. Now, no one could object when she hung out her nameplate: *Elizabeth Blackwell, M.D.*

Elizabeth continued to see patients in her office.

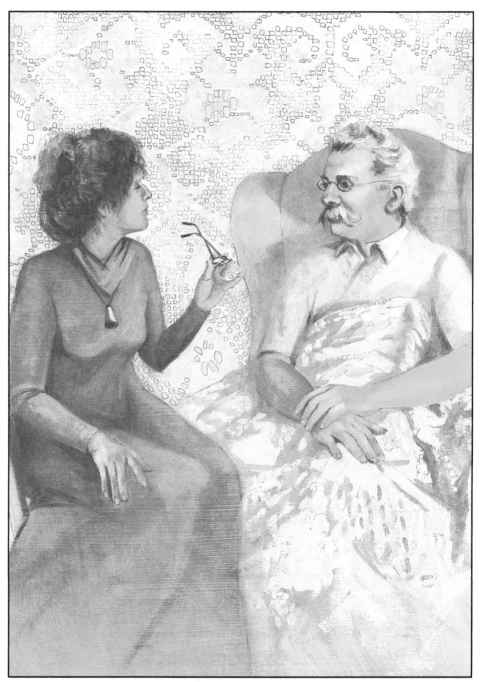

Word of Elizabeth's skill and kindness got around, and more patients came to trust the woman doctor. Often, she visited them in their homes.

And she ran the clinic by herself. She could call on other doctors to discuss her cases, but she wanted someone to work with her all the time. It would be years before Emily, who had gone to England to study, could join her.

One day, as if in answer to her wish, a young Polish woman stood at Elizabeth's door. Marie Zackrzewska had been a professor of midwives in a hospital in Berlin. Other doctors were jealous of her important position, and she was fired. In America to finish her education, she had heard about Dr. Blackwell, and hoped they could help each other.

All summer, the women worked side by side. Marie taught Elizabeth the latest practices in childbirth. Elizabeth taught Marie English and helped her get into medical school. When Marie left for school, Elizabeth was alone again. This time, she would not wait for a companion to find her. She would act on her own. Many children in the city had become orphans when their parents died of the epidemics so common among the poor. Elizabeth wanted to adopt one of these young girls and raise her as her daughter.

Kitty Barry was a thin, quiet seven-year-old when she came to live with Elizabeth. With good food, exercise, and a lot of attention, she became a bright, happy young girl. After a while, Dr. Emily Blackwell, then Dr. Marie Zackrzewska, joined them. Now the three doctors would work on yet another of Elizabeth's dreams. They would try to raise enough money to open a hospital for women run by women.

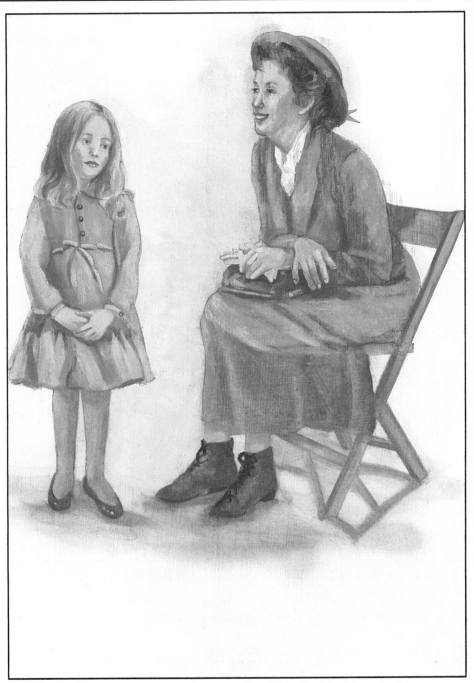

Elizabeth did not want to be alone again. She decided to adopt a poor girl whose parents had died in an epidemic.

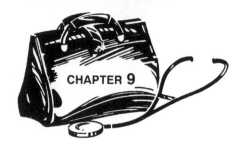

CHAPTER 9

Meeting the Challenge

On May 12, 1857, the New York Infirmary for
Women and Children — now New York Downtown
Hospital — was opened. Elizabeth picked that day —
Florence Nightingale's birthday — to honor her friend.
Florence had since become famous for treating
wounded British soldiers during the Crimean War.

Elizabeth was the director of the new hospital.
Emily was the surgeon, and Marie was the resident
doctor. Some patients visited the hospital's clinic
each day. Others had to stay in the hospital. People
who could afford to pay for treatment paid a small
amount. The poorest patients were treated free.

Within a month, all the beds were filled. Several
young women were being trained as nurses. The
doctors often worked from early morning until
midnight, breaking only for quick meals. Money
was always scarce, and they had to take in private
patients to keep up with expenses. There were
dangers in that first year, as well. After a woman
died from a fever, a crowd of her shouting relatives
and friends surrounded the hospital. *You in there!*

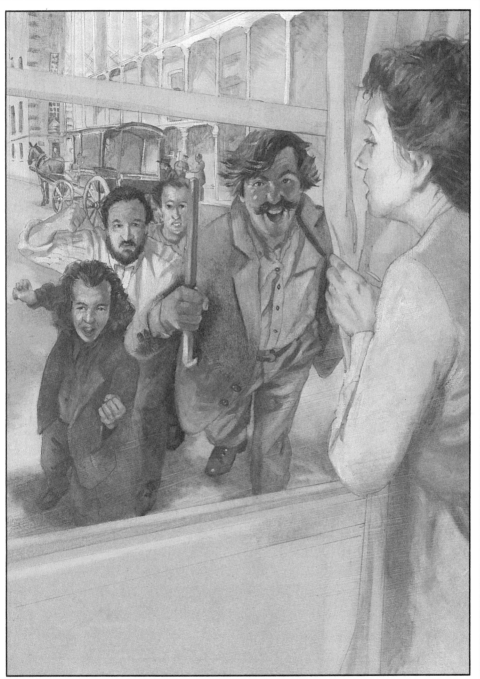

The angry crowd surrounded the hospital. Elizabeth watched from behind a curtain as a man with a crowbar approached the door.

Female doctors! Not doctors, killers! Kill women, that's what you do! We'll show you what we do to murderers!

As the crowd menaced the hospital, the three women tried to keep the patients calm. But locked doors and windows would be no protection if the angry mob tried to break in.

Suddenly, a man clutching a crowbar mounted the steps of the hospital. Elizabeth was ready to fling open the door and face the attack. But the man shouted above the crowd, "I ask you, what other doctors ever did as much for you? Gave you medicines, delivered your babies, cared whether you lived or died?" He was defending the hospital!

Ashamed of their actions, the people slowly turned and walked away. The hospital was safe. It could continue helping the people who so much needed help.

But the hospital, Elizabeth realized, was not enough. What about other women who wanted to become doctors? She would open a medical school so other women would not have to face the same obstacles she had faced. The school would need support and money. She thought she could get enough of both within a few years.

When the Civil War broke out in April 1861, plans for the school had to be put aside. It was more important now to train women to become nurses. These women would be sent to the various states of the Union to treat the thousands of men wounded in battle.

Slavery officially ended after the war. But women were still fighting for their rights. Again, Elizabeth started to line up supporters for her medical school.

At the same time, she worked out a system to bring health care into the community. She set up a team of "sanitary inspectors" to visit patients at home. The inspectors brought information on nutrition, child care, and cleanliness. Dr. Rebecca Cole, the first black woman doctor, was the head of the team for many years.

The Women's Medical College, a part of the New York Infirmary for Women and Children, opened in 1868. The school made Elizabeth proud. Many distinguished doctors agreed to be teachers. Others, like Elizabeth's friend Stephen Smith from Geneva, gave examinations to the students.

The first woman doctor in the United States had opened the nation's first medical school for other women. This would seem to be a fitting end to the efforts of Elizabeth Blackwell. But new challenges were still ahead.

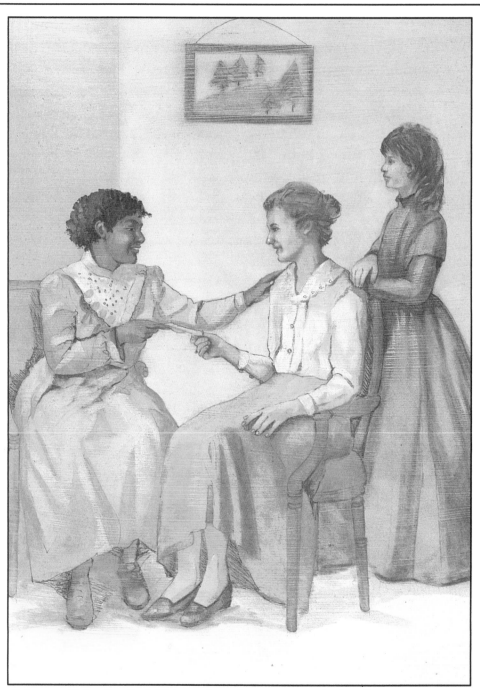

Rebecca Cole, the first African-American woman doctor, for many years headed a team of "sanitary inspectors" who visited patients at home.

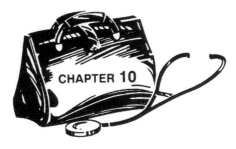

Looking Toward the Future

The medical profession was still closed to women in England. Elizabeth decided to leave her hospital. She would try to help women in England as she had helped women in America. "My work here is done," she told her sister Emily. "There's something in me that likes to start things anew. I guess I was born to be a pioneer."

In 1869, Elizabeth returned to the country where she was born. She set up a medical practice and sent for her daughter Kitty. As she had done in America, Elizabeth worked hard for important causes. She spoke about hygiene and child care. She lectured about the poor conditions in mines and factories. And she fought for the right of women to attend medical school. Her words were not popular with everyone.

But some women were inspired by Elizabeth's example to study medicine. Two of them, Elizabeth Garrett Anderson and Sophia Jex-Blake, got their degrees only after years of struggle against male opposition. In 1874, Elizabeth helped women establish the London School of Medicine for Women. She became a professor at the school, but she left after a few years because of poor health.

Although Elizabeth would not teach again, her voice was not silent. For the next 30 years, she worked to bring important ideas to the public. She spoke and wrote about hygiene and how it relates to disease prevention. She urged passage of laws against pollution. She wrote a book on sex education for young girls. At Kitty's urging, she wrote a book about her fight to become a doctor.

Family and friends were always welcome at Rock House, Elizabeth's home on the coast of England. Dr. Zackrzewska came with stories of her work in Boston. Like her friend, Marie had opened a hospital for women and children. And, also like Elizabeth, she had established a medical school to train women as doctors and nurses. Elizabeth and Marie recalled the past and wondered what the future would bring.

Would they have been surprised to learn that by the late twentieth century there were more than 80,000 women doctors in America? It surely would have pleased them to know that the opportunities in medicine had expanded in other ways, too. Today, medical careers include research, public health, and occupational health as well as private practice and nursing. And all areas are open to women.

Among the women who chose to be researchers are two who have received special honors. In 1977, Rosalyn Yalow shared the Nobel Prize for Medicine

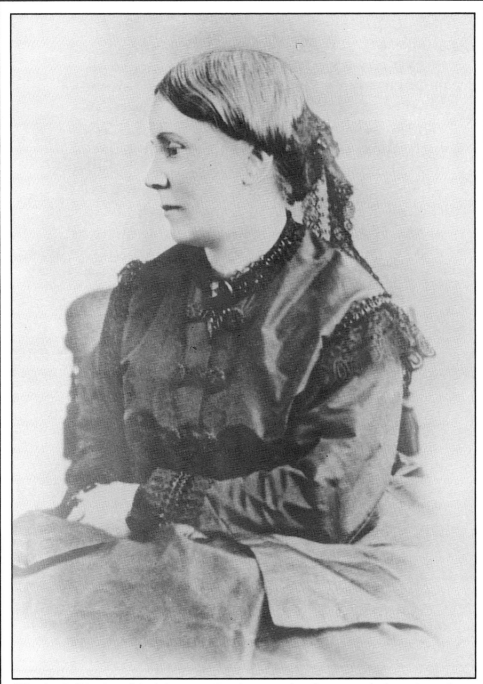

Elizabeth Blackwell led the way for thousands of women in her struggle to become America's first woman doctor.

with Roger Guillemin and Andrew Schally. They were recognized for their study of the role of hormones in the human body. In 1988, Gertrude Elion shared the Nobel Prize for Medicine with George Hitchings and James Black. Their research led to the development of new drugs to treat heart disease, leukemia, and other diseases.

Perhaps Elizabeth would have been most proud of another achievement — another first by a woman. In March of 1990, Dr. Antonia Novello became the first woman — and first Hispanic — Surgeon General of the United States. She thereby became the leading health adviser in the country. The job includes issuing warnings about public health dangers and setting up research on major health issues. The Surgeon General also works with other countries to solve worldwide health problems.

On May 31, 1910, Elizabeth Blackwell died at the age of 90. She had accomplished so much for herself. And, in doing so, she led the way for thousands of women who would follow her.

GLOSSARY

anatomy
(uh-NAT-uh-mee) the study of the structure of the human body

Crimean War
(kry-MEE-uhn wawr) a war (1853-1856) between Russia and Great Britain, France, Turkey, and Sardinia

dissect
(dihs-EHKT) to cut apart something to look at its structure

epidemic
(ehp-uh-DEHM-ihk) the spread of a disease to many people at once

hormone
(HAWR-mohn) chemicals made by the body that control the workings of some organs

hygiene
(HY-jeen) the science of the conditions and practices that help maintain good health

leukemia
(loo-KEE-mee-uh) a disease of the blood in which a large number of white blood cells are formed

midwife
(MIHD-wyf) a person who helps women give birth

missionary
(MIHSH-uh-nehr-ee) someone whose life is devoted to spreading a religion

philosophy
(fuh-LAHS-uh-fee) the study of beliefs and the reasons for them

presence
(PREHZ-ehns) the fact or condition of being present

quaint	(kwaynt) old-fashioned in a pleasing way
recommend	(rehk-uh-MEHND) to praise as worthy or good
reform	(rih-FAWRM) to change something in order to improve it
seamstress	(SEEM-struhs) a woman who makes her living by sewing
setback	(SEHT-bak) something that slows progress toward a goal
surgeon	(SUHR-juhn) a doctor who changes the body or removes diseased parts of the body by operation
tutor	(TOOT-uhr) someone who teaches privately, usually in a single subject
typhus	(TY-fuhs) a deadly disease, carried by body lice, marked by high fever, headaches, rashes, and a loss of mental control
Zackrzewska	(zah-KREHF-skah) Dr. Marie Zackrzewska, friend and partner of Elizabeth Blackwell